30 Days
Weight Loss Challenge

Conquer Cravings, Cultivate Balance, and Embrace a Healthier You in a 30-Day Journey.

By

Wesley L. Brodie

Table of Contents

INTRODUCTION

Are you prepared to set out on a path that will change not only your physical appearance but also the way you see health and wellbeing in general? Welcome to the "Weight Loss Challenge Spanning 30 Days"

Imagine living a life in which you can satisfy your cravings, eat the foods you love, achieve harmony in your daily schedule, and fully accept a healthier version of yourself. This book is meant to be your faithful ally on that journey; it is crafted to address the particular requirements, goals, difficulties, and preferences of people who are just like you.

It is simple to feel disoriented and discouraged in a world full of quick solutions and fad diets. Even though you may have danced with the concept of change, you were overwhelmed by the many steps and difficulties. We've experienced it.

We've all had the want for late-night snacks, been perplexed about what to eat, and yearned for long-lasting change.

This is the unique selling point of our 30-day challenge. Gaining control over your health, your relationship with food, and ultimately your life is more important than simply losing weight. The central figure in this adventure is you, our readers. We recognize that you're devoted exercise fanatics, time-pressed professionals, and health-conscious foodies. You're looking for a sustainable, well-rounded strategy since you've tried and failed.

Come along with us as we lead you toward conquering the cravings that have been holding you back for a very long time. You'll discover how to develop balance throughout your life, not only in your diet. Above all, you'll be equipped with the knowledge and skills necessary to genuinely accept a healthier version of yourself for the rest of your life, not just the next 30.

This book will provide you with individualized daily challenges, delicious recipes that you can enjoy guilt-free, true success stories, and useful tools to help you succeed on your journey. Now is the moment to take control of your health and live the life you've always wanted.

Turn the page and join me on this life-changing 30-day journey where you will develop balance, overcome cravings, and fully embrace the happier, healthier version of yourself that you have always wanted.

CHAPTER ONE

The 30-Day Weight Loss Challenge

Welcome to the 30-Day Weight Loss Challenge, the center of your life-changing adventure. This is where the magic happens, where you take major efforts toward becoming a healthier, happier version of yourself, and where your dreams are realized via doable actions.

We will accompany you for four weeks of commitment, resiliency, and self-exploration during this challenge. This trip has been carefully planned to not only help you lose excess weight but also to equip you with the skills and habits necessary to keep up your progress long after these 30 days are over.

A little peek at what's to come:

Week 1: Overcoming Addictions

We address cravings, one of the most frequent roadblocks to weight loss, in the first week. You'll discover which foods are your triggers, how to control your eating by practicing mindful eating, and how to stop those compulsive cravings by adopting healthy snacking habits.

Week 2: Developing Equilibrium

The secret to long-term weight loss is balance. In Week 2, we delve into the art of making nutrient-dense meals that fuel your body, learning how to plan meals, and balancing your macronutrients. You'll find that maintaining balance in your daily consumption doesn't need deprivation but rather a harmonious attitude.

Week 3: Adopting a Healthier Personality

This is the point where we treat your wellbeing as a whole. In Week 3, you'll develop stress management skills, prioritize sleep, and add exercise to your routine for a comprehensive wellness package. We'll walk you through monitoring your development so you can observe the amazing physical changes that are taking place.

Week 4: Maintaining Your Achievement

It's time to incorporate everything you've learned into your lifelong journey as the last week draws near. You'll keep up the healthy routines you've developed, reintroduce treats gradually without stopping your progress, and come up with long-term plans to guarantee long-lasting effects.

The 30-Day Weight Loss Challenge is about altering your relationship with food, exercise, and your lifestyle in general—it's not just about changing what you put on your plate. It's about taking back control of your health, escaping the never-ending cycle of dieting, and embracing a healthy version of yourself.

Prepare yourself to set out on this transformative journey. We'll overcome cravings, create balance, and, in the end, give you the confidence to accept a happier and healthier version of yourself. It's the beginning of a lifetime of wellbeing, not just 30 days.

Week 1: Overcoming Cravings

We take on one of the toughest opponents on the road to wellness in the first week of your 30-Day Weight Loss Challenge: cravings. It is common for cravings to feel like an overwhelming force, derail even the best-intentioned diet plans, and cause shame and frustration. The good news is that you can overcome cravings, and the first step on this empowering journey is to start in Week 1.

By the conclusion of the first week, you will have learned to embrace mindful eating, recognize your trigger foods, and lay the groundwork for a snacking strategy that is both healthful and nutritious. You'll be well on your way to managing your relationship with food, overcoming cravings, and forging a sustainable shift. The best is still to come in your 30-day metamorphosis, which is only getting started.

Identifying Food Triggers

The first step to taking back control of your eating habits in your quest for a better lifestyle is identifying and comprehending your trigger foods. Foods known as triggers are those delicious temptations that, once relished, can cause a wave of desires that eventually lead to overindulgence. It is difficult to avoid these foods since they frequently have strong emotional or psychological connections. Don't worry, though, because the first week of your 30-day weight loss challenge is devoted to assisting you in recognizing and managing these triggers.

The Power of Self-Awareness: Self-awareness is the starting point of the journey. You will engage in an introspective process to determine which foods are triggers for you. Think for a moment about your eating patterns. Which meals tend to make people overeat or make bad decisions? These could be salty nibbles, sweet delights, or even specific comfort foods. Embracing your vulnerabilities is the first step toward change.

Food Journaling: Maintaining a food journal is an effective way to identify trigger foods. Keep a journal of your daily meals and snacks, focusing on the times you felt pressured to overindulge. Note the items you ate, the conditions, and your feelings at the time. This journal turns into a reflection of your habits and tendencies, serving as a mirror for you.

Craving Patterns: We'll help you recognize trends in Week 1. Do you find that certain times of day are when cravings seem to occur? Are they brought on by social events, stress, or boredom? Knowing these tendencies gives you the ability to recognize and avoid circumstances that could encourage overindulgence.

Seeking Support: Never be afraid to ask friends, relatives, or a support group for assistance. Talk about the meals you're attempting to avoid as well as your journey. Finding and eliminating trigger foods can be greatly aided by the support and understanding of others.

Emotional Triggers: There's typically a connection between trigger foods and emotions. Think about the feelings causing your cravings. Are they associated with anxiety, melancholy, or joy? You can start looking for healthier, more alternative ways to deal with these emotions after you identify the emotional triggers.

You'll have a clear understanding of the things that trigger your desires by the conclusion of Week 1. Equipped with this understanding, you may proactively prevent or minimize these trigger meals for the remainder of your 30-day journey. One decision at a time, you are taking back control, and this is an essential step towards realizing your vision of overcoming cravings and embracing a healthier version of yourself.

Mindful Eating Practices

Your compass on the path to overcoming cravings and becoming a healthy version of yourself is mindful eating. It's a life-changing activity that focuses on how you eat and your relationship with food rather than just what you consume. During the first week of your 30-Day Weight Loss Challenge, you will learn this crucial skill that will help you become fully present in the moment and recover control over your eating patterns.

The Art of Being Completely Aware and Involved During Meals: This is the essence of mindful eating. It's about enjoying the sensory experience of eating, savoring every bite, and being aware of your body's hunger signals. A pleasant change from the norm is mindful eating in a society where eating is fast-paced and preoccupied.

Slowing Down: Reducing your speed is one of the first stages in mindful eating. Distractions such as televisions and cellphones should be put away, and your dining area should be calm. Enjoy your food's scents, tastes, and textures. You'll discover that doing this allows you to be satisfied with smaller servings.

Being Aware of Your Body's Signals: Eating mindfully helps you to develop an awareness of your body's signals. Do you eat because you're bored, stressed out, or are you genuinely hungry? Mindful eating is based on the understanding that physical hunger differs from emotional hunger.

The Factor of Satisfaction: Have you ever observed that your favorite dishes tend to taste best after the first few bites? You may identify this occurrence and enjoy those first few bites by practicing mindful eating. By following this technique, you can eat less and appreciate your food more.

Chew and Savor: Another essential element of mindful eating is chewing your meal well and appreciating every taste. You improve digestion and heighten your awareness of your body's fullness signals when you do this.

Remaining Present: Eating mindfully helps you to concentrate on your food and remain in the moment. It inhibits multitasking since it might cause inattention, which can result in overeating. Set aside time during meals to nurture your body and spirit.

You will incorporate these mindful eating techniques into your regular routine as you move through Week 1. The end result is a significant change in how you feel about eating, a renewed awareness of your body's natural cues, and an effective weapon for overcoming cravings. Adopting mindful eating will put you on the path to being a more aware and healthy version of yourself.

Optimal Snacking Techniques

We all snack occasionally, but it can either help you on your path to better health or become a roadblock. We discuss the art of healthy snacking in Week 1 of your 30-Day Weight Loss Challenge, giving you tips on how to squelch cravings, sustain your energy, and improve your general health.

Comprehending the Objective of Snacking: Snacks have to be a planned component of your regular diet rather than a guilty pleasure. Snacking is meant to sustain your energy levels, avoid severe hunger, which can result in overindulging, and supply vital nutrients to keep you full in between meals.

Wholesome Snack Options: Choose foods that are high in nutrients and low in empty calories. Opt for fresh fruits, vegetables, whole grains, lean protein sources, and healthy fats. These solutions give your body with important vitamins, minerals, and energy without needless additions or excessive sugar and salt.

Portion management: While nutritious snacks are a terrific choice, portion management is crucial. It's easy to overindulge in even the healthiest of snacks, which can lead to needless calorie intake. Use tiny containers or plates to limit servings and avoid mindlessly eating from a large bag or container.

Macronutrient Balancing: A combination of healthy fats, proteins, and carbs make up a balanced snack. This equilibrium prolongs your feeling of satisfaction and helps to maintain your blood sugar levels. For instance, think of combining Greek yogurt and berries or apple slices and almond butter.

Mindful Snacking: Make sure your snacking practices reflect the mindful eating guidelines you studied in Week 1. Eat your snacks mindfully, focusing on every bite, and without interruptions. By doing this, you'll be able to fully enjoy the flavor and satisfaction of your munchies.

Snacking on the Go: Having easy-to-graze, healthful alternatives on hand is crucial for people leading hectic lives. When you're out and about, pack healthy snacks like chopped vegetables, mixed nuts, or whole-grain crackers with hummus.

You'll have a variety of healthy snacking techniques at your disposal by the conclusion of the first week. These techniques will support you in overcoming cravings as well as sustaining consistent energy levels and proper dietary intake throughout the day. In order to become a healthier version of yourself, you must practice healthy snacking, which is something you can keep up long after your 30-day challenge is over.

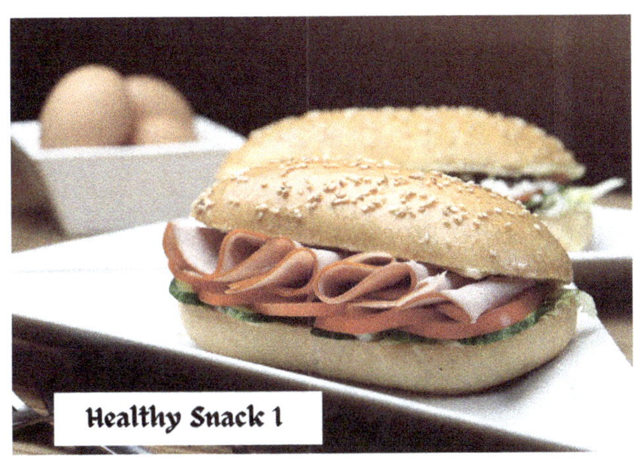

Healthy Snack 1

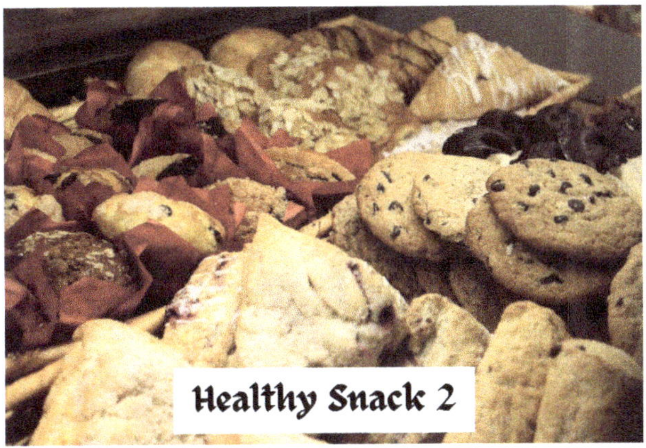

Healthy Snack 2

Week 2: Developing Equilibrium

Greetings and salutations for Week 2 of your 30-Day Weight Loss Challenge. As we continue on this life-changing path, we become more aware of the importance of balance. Maintaining a healthy and happy weight loss and overall well-being requires striking a balance between your diet, lifestyle, and general well-being.

Week 2 is all about creating a positive relationship with food and life, not just about nutrition. You're laying the groundwork for long-lasting improvement by developing nutrient-dense meals, learning how to balance macronutrients, and using efficient meal planning techniques. Embracing a better you for a lifetime of wellbeing, not simply for 30 days, starts this week.

Macro-Balancing in Meals

Macronutrient balancing, or eating meals that include the right amount of each macro, is a basic dietary principle that can significantly affect both your overall health and weight reduction efforts. Achieving your fitness and health objectives requires striking the correct balance between macronutrients, which are proteins, lipids, and carbs. We'll go into the practice of macro-balancing in Week 2 of your 30-Day Weight Loss Challenge, giving you a better knowledge of how to properly fuel your body.

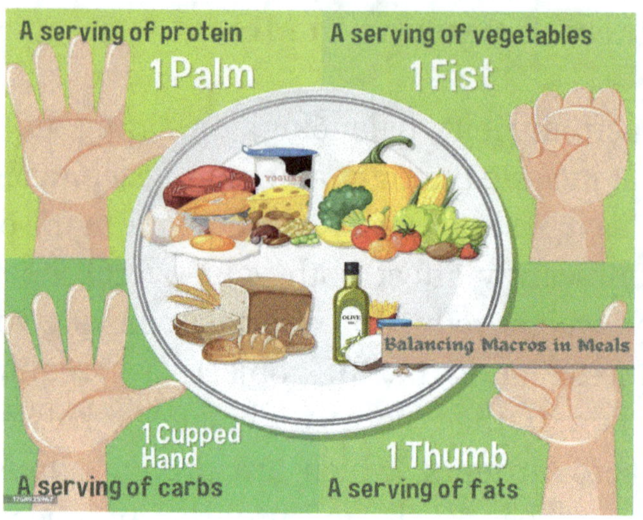

The Function of Carbohydrates: Your body uses carbohydrates as its main energy source. They supply the energy required for daily tasks, such as physical activity and cognitive processes. Nonetheless, selecting the appropriate varieties of carbs is crucial. We'll assist you in choosing complex carbs, which help to stabilize blood sugar levels and deliver energy gradually, such as whole grains, fruits, and vegetables.

The Value of Protein: Protein is your body's building block and is necessary for both muscular growth and tissue repair. Protein is essential for increasing fullness and decreasing cravings during meals. We'll discuss several lean protein sources, like fish, poultry, beans, and tofu, and how to include them in your diet to help you lose weight.

Recognizing Healthy Fats: Although fats have a poor rap, they are essential to good health. Nutrient absorption, brain function, and feeling full after eating are all significantly impacted by healthy fats, such as those in avocados, almonds, and olive oil. We'll show you how to choose healthy fats and include them into a diet that is well-balanced.

Discovering Your Perfect Balance: Everybody has a different optimum macro balance for their meals. Your ideal balance depends on things like age, exercise level, and special health objectives. We'll work with you to discover the ideal balance throughout Week 2 that suits your particular requirements.

Meal Planning with Macros in Mind: Having a well-thought-out meal plan gives you the ability to prepare meals that support your macro objectives. We'll go over useful tips and resources to help you organize wholesome, well-balanced meals that will help you on your path to being a healthier version of yourself.

Achieving a sustainable, balanced approach to nutrition is the goal of mealtime macro-balancing; it has nothing to do with severe dieting or restriction. You'll acquire the skills and self-assurance necessary to plan meals that complement your overall health and weight reduction objectives as you progress through Week 2. You may embrace a healthier and happier version of yourself by becoming an expert in the art of macronutrient balancing.

Formulating Recipes High in Nutrients

We switch gears in Week 2 of your 30-Day Weight Loss Challenge to developing nutrient-dense dishes. These dishes are meant to tantalize your taste buds while providing your body with necessary minerals, vitamins, and other nutrients. Nutrient-dense dishes are great because they allow you to eat well without compromising flavor.

The Nutrient-Dense Approach: Foods high in nutrients and low in calories are considered to be nutrient-dense. They give your body the nourishment it needs to grow and prosper. This week, you'll discover how to plan meals around these items so that you're eating for optimal health rather than just to feel satisfied.

Including a Range of Colors: Using a broad range of vibrant fruits and vegetables is one of the keys to developing nutrient-dense dishes. Consuming a rainbow of foods can guarantee that you get a wide range of vital vitamins and minerals, as different hues represent different nutritional values.

Selecting Lean Proteins: Nutrient-dense dishes must include lean proteins such skinless chicken, fish, tofu, and lentils. They provide muscle repair and maintenance with protein without being overly high in harmful saturated fats.

Healthy Fats: Well-balanced recipes use healthy fats, such as those in avocados, almonds, and olive oil, in a balanced way. Not only are these fats delightful, but they are also essential for brain function, long-lasting fullness, and the absorption of nutrients.

Whole Grains and Fiber: Whole grains offer vital fiber that supports a healthy digestive system and feeling full. Examples of these are brown rice, quinoa, and whole wheat pasta. These grains are embraced by nutrient-dense dishes, which guarantee satisfying and fulfilling meals.

Flavor and Health: Adding herbs and spices to your food can enhance its flavor and provide additional health advantages. You may improve the flavor and add additional layers of nutrients and antioxidants to your meals by adding spices like turmeric, garlic, and rosemary.

Tailoring for Your Requirements: In Week 2, you will receive guidance on developing nutrient-dense dishes that meet your specific dietary needs and tastes. You'll be able to change recipes to fit your preferences and still adhere to your health objectives.

When you explore the world of nutrient-dense meals, you'll find that eating well can be tasty and enjoyable. These recipes will help you lose weight while also bringing fresh vigor and vitality into your daily existence. Making scrumptious and nourishing meals that feed your body from the inside out this week is an exciting start toward adopting a healthier you.

How to Plan Meals for Success

In the second week of the 30-Day Weight Loss Challenge, meal preparation is your hidden weapon. With the help of this effective tool, you can take charge of your nutrition and make sure that your meals support your objectives for a happier, healthier you. Achieving long-term weight loss requires effective meal planning, which sets the stage for success by integrating healthy eating into your daily schedule in a simple and manageable manner.

Why Is Meal Planning Important? The daily grind can frequently result in impulsive, unhealthy eating decisions. Planning your meals will help you avoid this frequent mistake. You position yourself for success if you take the effort to prepare your meals once a week. Having wholesome options close at hand will lessen the urge to eat poorly on a whim.

Macro and nutrient balancing is made possible by meal planning, which enables you to do just that. You can make sure that every meal helps you achieve your weight loss objectives and maintain general health by carefully choosing your proteins, carbs, and healthy fats.

Variety and Satisfaction: Well-thought-out meal preparation guarantees a range of tastes and cuisines. Healthy eating is more pleasurable and sustainable when there is diversity. Your taste buds will appreciate it, and you'll look forward to your meals.

Meal planning has several advantages, one of which is portion control. Preparing your meals in advance helps you control your calorie intake and avoid overindulging. A key component of effective weight loss is this.

Reduced Food Waste: By assisting you in purchasing and preparing only what you need, meal planning helps you reduce food waste. It's an economical, environmentally friendly method that improves the environment and your health.

Streamlined Shopping: A carefully planned menu makes food shopping a snap.

Knowing exactly what you need will make shopping trips easier and less impulsive buys.

Meal planning provides flexibility and adaptability. Your plans can be modified to fit your preferences and schedule. With the help of this application, you can maintain your progress toward your health objectives even on the busiest of days.

We'll help you create efficient meal plans in Week 2 that suit your dietary requirements, tastes, and macro objectives. You'll have a customized meal planning technique by the end of the week that facilitates your weight loss efforts and makes eating healthily easier. Meal planning is a life skill that will help you on your journey to a better, happier you. It's not just a skill for this 30 days.

Week 3: Adopting a Healthier Personality

Now that Week 3 of your 30-Day Weight Loss Challenge has arrived, it's time to commit to a comprehensive plan for a healthier you. This week is about taking care of your mind and spirit in addition to your physical health. We'll explore the behaviors and ideas that result in a life that is more contented and balanced.

A crucial stage in your quest for a healthier you is week three. You're taking crucial steps toward living a healthy and fulfilled life by combining exercise, controlling stress, prioritizing sleep, and keeping track of your progress. This week is dedicated to promoting your mental and emotional well-being, which will enable you to reach your full potential as a person, in addition to your physical health. If you adopt this all-encompassing strategy, you'll be well on your way to being a happier, healthier version of yourself.

Including Exercise in Your Daily Routine

This week on your 30-Day Weight Loss Challenge, we're going to introduce you to exercise—one of the mainstays of a healthier you. On your path to wellbeing, incorporating regular physical activity into your daily routine is a game-changing move. Let's look at some methods for incorporating fitness into your life that you can stick with and enjoy.

Discovering Your Fitness Passion: Exercising should be fun and something you look forward to, not a chore. Discovering your passion is the first step towards adopting exercise. Find anything that you enjoy doing, whether it's yoga, dancing, swimming, or running. Enjoying what you do makes it more than a job; it becomes a way of life.

Establishing Realistic Goals: Start with attainable objectives. Excessive expectations can cause dissatisfaction and a lack of motivation. As your fitness improves, start with reasonable expectations and progressively raise the duration and intensity of your workouts.

Making a Schedule: It's essential to plan out your workouts. Exercise should be approached with the same level of dedication as any other appointment. Schedule your workouts at precise times, and try your best to keep to it. Success comes from being consistent.

Cross-training and Variety: Mix things up in your workout regimen. This keeps things interesting and helps you avoid overuse injuries and progress plateaus. Think about mixing up your strength training, flexibility, and cardiovascular regimens.

Accountability and Support: Occasionally, enrolling in a fitness class or finding a workout partner might give you the accountability and drive you need. You can stay on track and enjoy the exercise routine more when you exercise with others.

Gradual Progression: Don't jump right into hard training. A gradual increase lowers the chance of harm and lets your body adjust. As you gain confidence and fitness, gradually increase the intensity of your routines from a comfortable starting point.

Celebrate Milestones: Acknowledge and honor your accomplishments as you go forward. Acknowledging your achievements, whether they be from jogging an extra mile, lifting bigger weights, or perfecting a yoga pose, helps you stay motivated and goal-focused.

Including exercise in your routine will help you build strength, vitality, and overall well-being in addition to helping you lose weight. You can achieve a healthy you by engaging in activities you enjoy, establishing reasonable goals, making a routine, and trying out different types of exercise. Exercise benefits not only your physical health but also your mental and emotional well-being, quality of life, and equilibrium in your overall wellbeing.

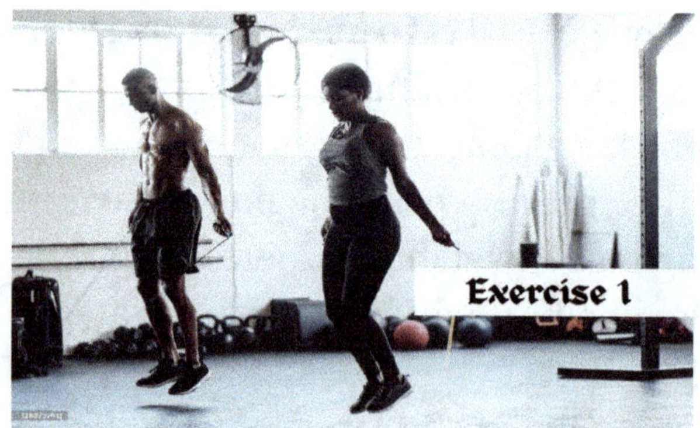

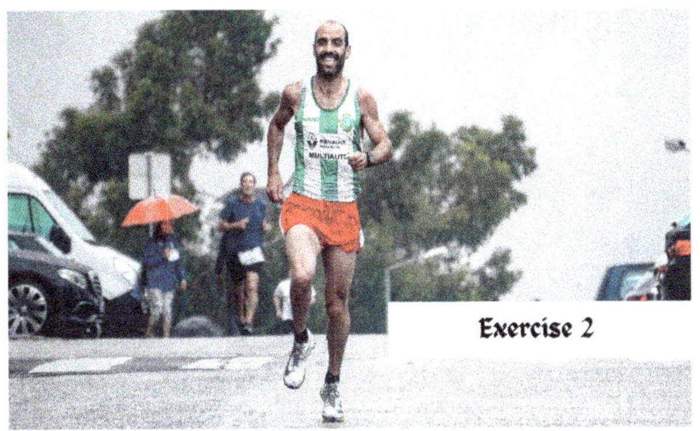

Stress Reduction and Proper Sleep Practices

We go into two essential components of holistic health in Week 3 of your 30-Day Weight Loss Challenge: stress management and sleep hygiene. These are frequently disregarded elements that significantly affect your entire well-being, including your efforts to lose weight. Let's look at methods for reducing stress and enhancing sleep quality.

Stress management: Although stress is a normal aspect of modern life, prolonged stress can harm your health and undermine your attempts to lose weight. Here's how to efficiently handle it:

Meditation and Mindfulness: Schedule time each day for meditation and mindfulness. By engaging in these activities, you can improve your emotional health, lessen worry, and remain in the present.

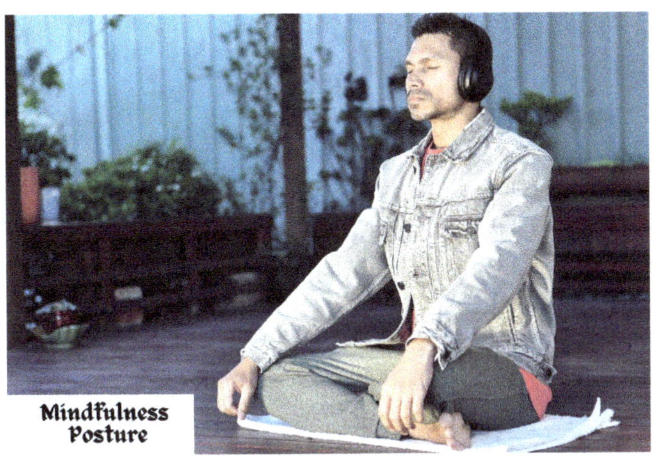

Mindfulness
Posture

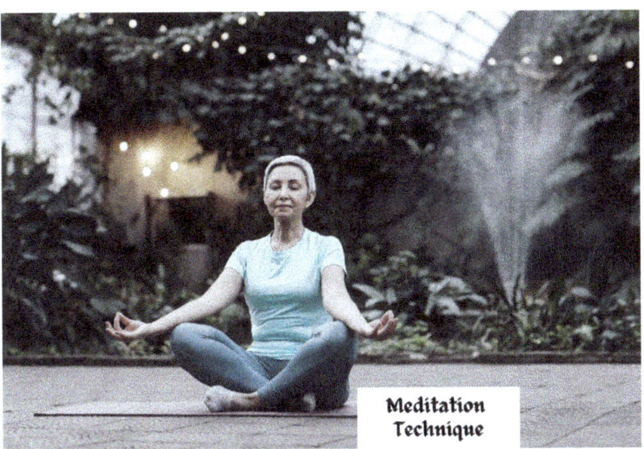

Meditation
Technique

Physical Activity: Exercising on a regular basis not only improves your physical health but also effectively reduces stress. It causes endorphins, which are your body's natural mood enhancers, to be released.

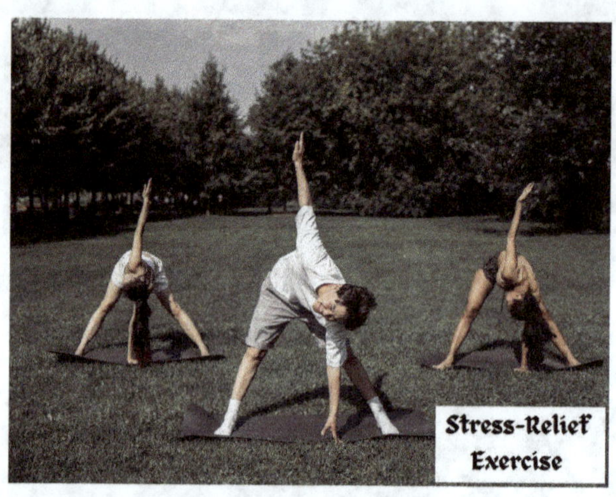

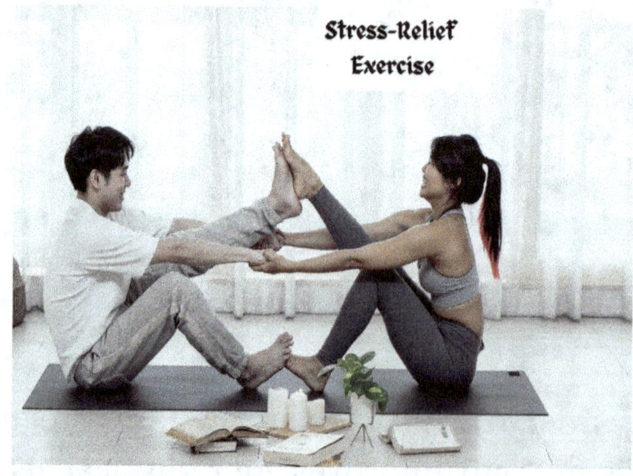

Breathing Techniques: You can instantly relax with deep breathing techniques, which you may perform anywhere. Use these techniques to help you de-stress and ease tension when you're feeling anxious.

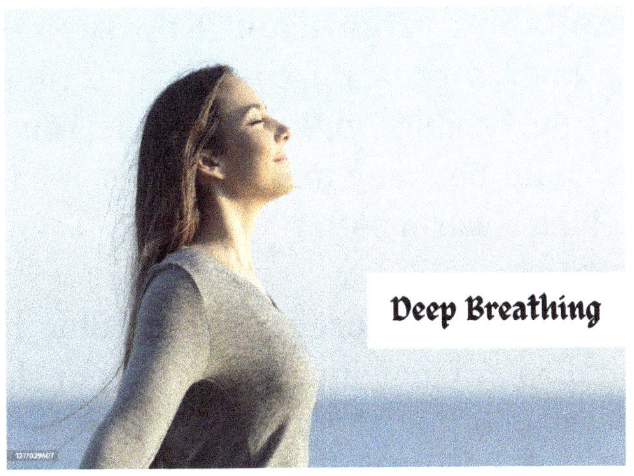

Time management involves setting priorities and organizing your workload. Stress is decreased by a well-planned day because it gives you a sense of control over your obligations.

Sleep hygiene: Getting enough sleep is critical for weight loss, mental clarity, and overall wellness. Hormones that control appetite and hunger can be upset by sleep deprivation, which can result in weight gain. Here's how to enhance your quality of sleep:

Establish a nighttime Routine: Give your body a constant cue that it's time to sleep by establishing a nighttime routine. This could be doing mild stretches, reading, or taking a warm bath.

Cut Down on Screen Time: Blue light from displays may interfere with your sleep. At least one hour before going to bed, stay away from screens of any kind, including TVs, phones, and tablets.

Optimize Your Sleep Environment: Make sure your bedroom is cold, quiet, and dark. Purchase pillows and a comfortable mattress.

Limit Alcohol and Caffeine: Because they can disrupt your sleep patterns, avoid alcohol and caffeine right before bed.

Control Stress: As was already mentioned, reducing stress is essential to getting a better night's sleep. Using stress management practices might improve your sleep quality indirectly, as stress can cause insomnia and disturbed sleep.

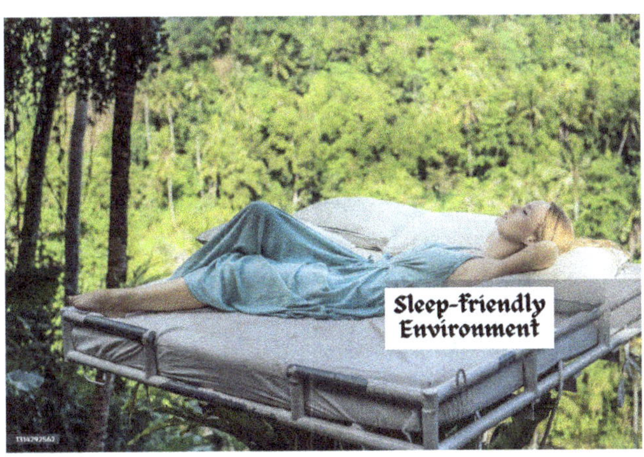

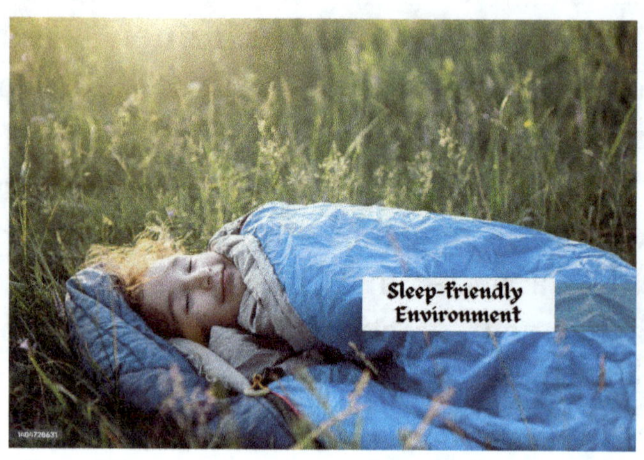

You are taking vital measures to guarantee your general health and well-being by becoming an expert in stress management and sleep hygiene. These habits will improve the quality of your life in addition to aiding in your weight loss attempts. In order to become a healthier, happier version of yourself, week three is all about finding balance in all facets of your life. Reducing stress and enhancing sleep quality are key components of this.

Monitoring Progress

Self hit a turning point in your 30-Day Weight Loss Challenge during Week 3, when keeping track of your progress becomes crucial to your quest for a healthy self. Tracking involves more than just keeping an eye on your weight; it also involves evaluating how your physical and emotional health have changed, celebrating your accomplishments, and maintaining your will to keep going.

Establishing Clear measurements: It's critical to set clear measurements in order to monitor your development efficiently. This surpasses the scale's numerical value. Take into account variables such as physical endurance, mood, energy levels, body measurements, and even non-scale successes like getting back into an old pair of clothes or having less cravings.

Using Technology: You can track your progress with a variety of wearables and apps. In addition to many other data, they can track heart rate, daily steps, sleep quality, and more. By using these resources, you can gain insightful knowledge about your journey.

Taking Before and After Pictures: These images are an effective visual aid for monitoring development. They can offer a concrete documentation of your metamorphosis, which can inspire you when you realize how far you've come.

Keeping a Journal: You can keep track of your daily routine, feelings, and thoughts by keeping a progress journal. This enables you to spot trends and adjust appropriately.

Frequent Weigh-Ins: Although the weight on the scale is only one factor to consider, tracking your weight reduction progress with regular weigh-ins can be insightful. But keep in mind that everyday variances are common, so don't let little differences depress you.

Milestone Celebration: No matter how minor your accomplishments may seem, acknowledge and appreciate them as you monitor your development. Acknowledging and rewarding oneself for your efforts can be an effective source of motivation.

Remaining Consistent: When it comes to monitoring your development, consistency is essential. Whether you plan to track on a daily, weekly, or monthly basis, establish a regular regimen. By being consistent, you can be confident that the record of your travel is accurate.

Modifying Your strategy: As you monitor your development, you can identify areas in which your strategy needs to be modified. Use the information you collect to fine-tune your strategy, whether it be your stress management strategies, food choices, or exercise regimen.

You can learn a lot about your journey by keeping a detailed log of your progress. You'll be able to clearly see your achievements as well as your areas for improvement. This information gives you the ability to stay focused, stay inspired, and eventually accept a better version of yourself. Taking control of your health is the focus of week three, and monitoring your development is essential to reaching this objective.

Week 4: Maintaining Your Achievement

The emphasis of your 30-Day Weight Loss Challenge will now be on maintaining your progress and making the switch to a longer-term, healthier lifestyle as you approach Week 4. This week is all about ensuring that the positive adjustments you've made are permanent, keeping up your progress, and reinforcing the habits you've formed.

In addition to marking the end of your 30-Day Weight Loss Challenge, Week 4 marks the start of your ongoing quest for wellbeing. Making sustainable, balanced, introspective, and goal-oriented changes will help you make sure that the improvements you've made stay in your life. Accept the lessons you've learnt and use them to maintain your wellbeing. The journey to a healthy you is a continuous one, but with the skills and information you've acquired, you can make it a worthwhile and long-lasting one.

Reintroducing Treats Gradually

One of the most important things to remember in Week 4 of your 30-Day Weight

Loss Challenge is to gradually start reintroducing treats. This idea highlights how important it is to maintain a healthy lifestyle while indulging in your favorite foods in a mindful and balanced manner. The following is an effective way to handle this reintroduction:

Mindful Approach: Mindfulness is the key to the methodical reintroduction of sweets. It's about really appreciating your indulgences rather than overindulging or putting restrictions on yourself. You can eat your favorite meals and still be in control if you do this.

Setting Boundaries: Specify parameters in detail before reintroducing treats. This entails choosing the frequency and amount of your indulgence. Establishing limits keeps your goodies in moderation and helps avoid overindulgence.

Quality Above Quantity: Prioritize quality over quantity while indulging in sweets. Select confections that genuinely satiate your appetite and delight your taste buds. Instead of mechanically consuming more inferior goods in increasing quantities, savor every bite.

Maintaining a Balance: While reintroducing treats, make sure they are balanced with nutrient-dense meals and snacks. This guarantees that your total diet stays in line with your health objectives. Treats should be viewed as a rare complement to a diet that is primarily healthy.

Planned Treats: Take into account setting aside particular days or events for treats. This may be a monthly trip to your preferred restaurant or a weekly dessert night. Setting up a routine helps you to prepare ahead and avoid impulsive indulgence.

Relishing Without Guilt: It's critical to relish your sweets guilt-free. An unhealthy relationship with eating might result from guilt. Recall that snacks can be safely enjoyed without impeding your progress, as they are a regular part of life.

Exercise and Balance: You can counteract indulgences if you're worried about how they might affect your weight. Just be sure to get more exercise. On treat days, you can counteract the extra calories with a longer walk or an extra activity.

One of the most important steps in maintaining your success after the 30-Day Challenge is to gradually reintroduce goodies. It's a skill that gives you the ability to live a full, balanced life without feeling inadequate. You may enjoy the odd indulgence and maintain your commitment to a better you by indulging in pleasures with awareness and intention.

Sustaining Well-Being Behaviors

The emphasis of Week 4 of your 30-Day Weight Loss Challenge is on making the switch from a short-term to a long-term effort. The secret to making sure the good adjustments you've made last the rest of your life is to keep up the healthy routines you've developed. The following are some practical methods for keeping up these habits:

Remaining consistent is essential to sustaining healthy habits. Your 30-Day Challenge has taught you many valuable habits that you should incorporate into your daily routine, whether they have to do with sleep, stress management, nutrition, or exercise. Try to follow these routines every day with consistency.

Establish Realistic Goals: You don't have to keep up the same pace and intensity as you did during the challenge to continue on your path to a healthy you. Make fresh long-term goals that are doable. These could be benchmarks like covering a set distance in running, holding onto a given weight, or reaching a particular degree of stress reduction.

Plan and Prioritize: Make daily habit plans in the same way that you have planned your meals and exercise during the challenge. Prioritize your well-being, schedule time for exercise, and prepare meals. It's been said that failing to plan is planning to fail.

Remain Accountable: Remaining accountable is a great way to keep up good practices. Whether it's a friend, relative, or a support group, let them know about your ambitions. They can encourage you when things get hard and help you stay on course.

Learn from Difficulties: Be prepared for obstacles and failures when traveling.

Consider them as chances to develop and learn, rather than as failures. What led to the failure, and how can you avoid repeating the same mistakes in the future?

Celebrate your accomplishments as a self-reward. When you accomplish your goals, reward yourself and recognize your accomplishments. Incentives might motivate you to keep up your healthy routines.

Seek Professional Guidance: To assist you in upholding healthy behaviors, think about seeking advice from experts in the field, such as a therapist, personal trainer, or nutritionist. Their knowledge can offer insightful advice and direction.

Being flexible is essential because life is dynamic and routines may need to modify from time to time. Be adaptable when it comes to changing your routines and

making sure they still support your health
objectives.

You may make sure that the beneficial
adjustments you've made to your lifestyle
stick by continuing to practice the healthy
habits you developed during the challenge.
It's about the lifelong road to a healthier,
happier self, not just a 30-day makeover.
You'll achieve long-term success and
wellbeing if you can maintain these
practices.

CHAPTER TWO

Personalized Challenges

We introduce the idea of tailored challenges in Week 4 of your 30-Day Weight Loss Challenge. Customization is an effective strategy to make sure that your road toward health and fitness is a customized one that meets your own needs, tastes, and goals rather than just a one-size-fits-all one.

Creating personalized challenges is a way to personalize your health journey. You're making a path that fits your life by focusing on your specific requirements, addressing your challenges, including what you love, and setting your own pace. Week 4 is about starting a lifelong road to well-being that is uniquely tailored to you, not merely finishing a 30-day challenge. Accept the obstacles that are unique to you and enjoy the journey to a better, happier version of yourself.

Daily Challenges

The foundation of your road to a better you are everyday struggles. Even though your 30-Day Weight Loss Challenge is almost over, the idea of daily challenges guarantees that you will keep improving and developing every day. These challenges are tiny, doable actions you perform every day to establish and uphold your healthy routines. Daily challenges can help you in the following ways:

Daily challenges center on the development of habits and consistency. You can strengthen your good habits by making a daily commitment to a small, health-related task. Building habits requires consistency, which is why everyday challenges help you maintain your routines.

Daily challenges place an emphasis on progress rather than perfection. It's not necessary to make big announcements or significant adjustments every day. Rather, concentrate on tiny, doable actions that eventually result in a steady development.

Concentrate on Specific Objectives: Daily challenges can be adapted to certain objectives or areas in which you hope to make progress. These daily objectives, which range from drinking more water to eating more veggies to walking for an additional ten minutes each day, are focused and productive.

Daily Challenges: Mindful Living is Encouraged. You become more present in your daily life when you make daily aims and act to fulfill them. This awareness encompasses your daily routines for exercise, food, and general wellbeing.

Increased Accountability: Having a daily task to do makes you more accountable. Even on the busiest or most difficult days, you can stay on course with the support of this accountability.

Celebrating Everyday Success: You can have everyday celebrations of your accomplishments by establishing and accomplishing daily tasks. These modest successes can increase your self-worth and motivation.

Flexibility and Adaptability: Everyday obstacles can be modified to fit your particular situation. If you have a very busy day, your challenge might be as easy as taking a few minutes to practice deep breathing. You might have more ambitious plans for other days. Its adaptability guarantees that you can take part at all times.

Long-Term Commitment: Your long-term dedication to health is supported by daily challenges. They are for life, not only for thirty days. Your health journey will be long-lasting if you incorporate everyday challenges into your continuing lifestyle.

Your journey to become a healthy version of yourself must include daily challenges. They are the little actions you take every day that, when combined, produce big results. Accept daily challenges as a tool for ongoing development, habit reinforcement, and mindful living as you move past your 30-Day Challenge. Recall that in the end, it's the little things that add up to the most.

Weekly Challenge Samples

Organizing your daily tasks into weekly themes with a distinct focus is one of the best ways to incorporate them into your life. Taking this method guarantees a comprehensive and well-rounded path to a healthy you, while also keeping your everyday difficulties engaging. Weekly themes are used to arrange these sample challenges into weekly categories:

"Foundation of Wellness" is the theme for Week 1.

Example of Challenge:

Day 1: Challenge of Hydration
Try to consume 64 ounces, or at least 8 glasses, of water today.

Day 2: Eating Consciously

Today, eat just one meal, paying attention to every bite.

Day 3: Every Day Jog
Today, make time for a 15-minute stroll. Make use of this time to decompress.

Day 4: Swap Healthful Snacks
Choose a healthier snack instead of your usual one, like nuts or fruit.

Day 5: Journal of Gratitude
Make a list of the three things you are grateful for today.

Week two: "Physical Activity and Movement"

Example of Challenge:

Day 1: Daily Stretching
Stretch for ten minutes to start your day.

Day 2: Heart Day
Set aside twenty minutes for a cardiovascular exercise regimen (such as a brisk walk, jog, or jump rope).

Day 3: Exercise with Strength
Spend fifteen minutes doing bodyweight workouts like squats and push-ups.

Day 4: Recuperation and Rest
Use mild yoga or deep breathing techniques to concentrate on relaxation.

Day 5: Nature Exploration
Take an hour to explore a local park, go bicycling, or go on a hike.

Week three: "Mindfulness and Stress Reduction"

Example of Challenges:

Day1: Meditation in the morning
Set a tranquil tone for the day by starting with a 10-minute meditation practice.

Day 2: Walk of Gratitude
While you stroll, concentrate on the things for which you are thankful.

Day 3: De-stressing Pause
Take a five-minute break to practice deep breathing whenever you feel stressed.

Day 4: Holistic Reset
Before going to bed, unplug from screens for at least an hour.

Day 5: Evening Thoughts
Before going to bed, put your ideas down on paper and consider the events of the day.

The fourth week's topic is "Balanced Lifestyle".

Example of Challenges

Day 1: Equilibrium Dish Combine vegetables, nutritious grains, and lean protein to create a well-balanced dinner.

Day 2: Customized Exercise
Create an exercise program that suits your tastes and fitness objectives.

Day 3: Introspective Relishment
Savor a little treat, paying attention to each bite.

Day 4: Charitable Deeds
Throughout the day, commit three random acts of kindness.

Day 5: Making Future Plans
Establish clear long-term objectives for your journey toward health and fitness.

These weekly example challenges give your daily challenges structure and make sure you cover a range of wellness and health topics. You are welcome to modify and customize these tasks to fit your own requirements and tastes, making them a fun and long-lasting component of your ongoing commitment to wellbeing.

Tailoring Difficulties to Personal Preferences

The adaptability and flexibility of daily tasks is one of their main advantages. Making your wellness path uniquely yours requires that you adapt obstacles to your own tastes. You can modify daily tasks to suit your requirements and tastes in the following ways:

Define Your Objectives: Start by outlining your objectives for wellness and health. What goals are you aiming to accomplish? Knowing what your goals are—be it stress relief, better sleep, weight loss, or fitness—is the first step toward overcoming everyday obstacles.

Customize Fitness Challenges: If improving your fitness is your main objective, modify daily tasks by concentrating on enjoyable pursuits. Include dancing in your everyday routine if you enjoy it. Incorporate challenges based on yoga if you enjoy the calm style of yoga. Tailoring workout challenges to your own needs will keep you interested and inspired.

Respect Dietary Preferences: It's important to modify dietary restrictions based on personal preferences. Focus on nutrition challenges that are plant-based if you are a vegetarian or vegan. Adapt your challenges to meet your unique needs if you have food restrictions or allergies. Making a food plan that suits your eating preferences is crucial.

Stress Management Personalized for You: If stress management is the main source of your everyday issues, then modify them to fit your chosen methods of stress reduction. Select hobbies or pastimes that you enjoy, such as art, music, journaling, or meditation. This guarantees that the tasks aimed at reducing stress will actually help you.

Personalized Self-Care: Self-care tasks must to be made in accordance with your personal inclinations. Adapt your self-care tasks to activities that support your well-being, whether that means reading, taking long walks in nature, going to the spa, or just enjoying some quiet time for introspection.

Pick the Right Time: Take into account your everyday obligations and timetable. If you find that the mornings are too busy for your difficulties, rearrange them to fit into a more comfortable time of day. Timing flexibility makes it possible for you to regularly overcome obstacles.

Personalized Accountability: Customize your accountability framework to align with your individual style. While some people prefer a more solitary approach, others flourish in a community setting. Pick the accountability method that works best for you, whether it's telling friends, family, or a mentor about your accomplishments.

Celebrate Your Individual route: Keep in mind that you have a unique route to wellbeing. Accept your uniqueness and acknowledge your advancements. Adapt daily challenges to suit your pace and style. Realize that you have a unique journey to a healthy self, and you should be proud of that.

Tailoring challenges to personal preferences enhances the enjoyment and sustainability of your wellness journey. It makes sure that the daily tasks you set for yourself are consistent with your goals, preferences, and way of life, allowing them to become an essential part of your everyday routine. You're not just getting healthier by personalizing your difficulties; you're also experiencing the happiness and fulfillment that come from following a route that is especially made for you.

CHAPTER THREE

Delicious And Guilt-Free Recipes

Redefining your connection with food is a crucial step on your path to becoming a healthier version of yourself. The misconception that eating healthily is boring or unfulfilling is completely untrue. We introduce you to delectable, guilt-free foods in Week 4 of your 30-Day Weight Loss Challenge that will satisfy your palate as well as your body.

Making the switch to a healthier diet doesn't mean giving up flavor or satisfaction. Recipes that are delicious and guilt-free will change the way you think about food. They keep you on track with your fitness and health objectives while transforming meals into pleasurable experiences. Proving that you can have your cake—or a healthy version of it—and eat it too is the focus of week four. Accept these recipes and allow them to inspire you to become a better, happier version of yourself via the pleasure of attentive, delectable eating.

Recipes to Beat Cravings

One of the biggest steps in becoming a healthy version of yourself is overcoming cravings. Food cravings that are unhealthy, sweet, or rich in calories have the tendency to impede your development. We introduce you to craving-conquering meals in Week 4 of your 30-Day Weight Loss Challenge, which will help you not only control these strong cravings but also offer a wholesome and tasty substitute. Here's how incorporating these recipes into your diet could revolutionize it:

Intelligent ingredient substitutions are used in the creation of dishes that beat cravings. They swap out unhealthy or high-calorie components for wholesome substitutes that satiate your appetites without sacrificing your objectives.

Desserts to Consider: These dishes provide guilt-free options for those with a sweet taste. Savor a delightful dessert while controlling your sugar intake. Desserts don't have to be unhealthy—as demonstrated by these dishes, which include chocolate avocado mousse and berry parfait.

Protein-R-Packed Snacks: Between meals, cravings frequently arise. These dishes offer high-protein snacks that satisfy your hunger and help you control it. You can easily suppress your appetite by snacking on foods like roasted chickpeas or Greek yogurt with fruit.

Makeovers for Comfort Food: Comfort foods can include a lot of calories and bad fats. Recipes that satisfy cravings reimagine traditional favorites in a healthier way.
Savor comfortable yet incredibly healthful foods like cauliflower crust pizza or zucchini noodles with tomato sauce.

Savory Satisfaction: There are dishes that satiate the cravings of people who are in the mood for savory flavors. These healthful recipes, which range from baked sweet potato fries to homemade veggie burgers, are flavorful and full of umami.

Baking with mindfulness: If you enjoy baking, check out these recipes for healthier substitutions that don't sacrifice flavor. Make healthy ingredient-focused baked products such as wholegrain muffins, pancakes made with almond flour, or brownies with black beans.

Quantity management: A key component of recipes that combat cravings is quantity management. They give you just enough to satiate your appetites without going overboard.

Sustainable Solutions: By emphasizing whole, minimally processed products, these recipes prioritize sustainable eating. They enhance your wellbeing and encourage environmentally beneficial decisions.

Choosing carefully is the key to beating cravings, not restriction. Recipes that combat cravings allow you to indulge in your favorite flavors without sacrificing your commitment to wellbeing and health. By making these meals a part of your regular routine, you're doing more than simply controlling cravings—you're also acknowledging your accomplishments and enjoying eating for a better you.

Healthy, Well-Rounded Meals

A healthier you starts with meals that are nutrient-rich and well-balanced. We introduce you to these meals in Week 4 of your 30-Day Weight Loss Challenge; they taste fantastic, support overall wellbeing, and supply you with vital nutrients. Here's how nutrient-dense, well-balanced meals can change the way you think about nutrition:

Comprehensive Nutrition: You can get a variety of vital nutrients from well-balanced and nutrient-rich meals, such as vitamins, minerals, healthy fats, proteins, and carbs. They promote your general wellbeing and health.

Satisfying and Filling: The goal of these meals is to provide both satisfaction and nourishment. To help you feel full and avoid overeating, they mix the proper ratios of macronutrients including protein, fiber, and good fats.

Delicious Variation: This is one of the main features of these dishes. They combine a variety of flavors, ingredients, and cooking techniques. This diversity guarantees that you get a range of nutrients and also makes your meals interesting.

Portion Control: A key component of well-balanced, nutrient-rich meals is moderation. They give you sensible portion sizes so you may eat good meals without going overboard.

Tailored to Preferences: These dishes can be adjusted to meet your dietary needs and constraints. You can modify these dishes to fit your dietary requirements, whether you're a vegetarian, vegan, gluten-free, or adhere to another diet.

Meal Planning Made Simple: Nutrient-rich, well-balanced meals make meal planning simple for people with hectic schedules. They give you a recipe for well-balanced, healthful food, making planning and preparation easier.

Sustainable Eating: By emphasizing complete, minimally processed foods, these dishes place a high priority on sustainability. They promote environmentally sustainable decisions and a more mindful eating style.

Mindful Eating: Nutrient-dense, well-balanced meals promote mindful eating. They encourage paying attention to your body's signals of hunger and fullness, enjoying the flavors of your food, and being mindful of the moment when you eat.

Weight management: You can modify these meals to meet your own goals, regardless of whether you're trying to gain, maintain, or reduce weight. They give you options that are balanced and portion managed, which makes it easier for you to efficiently manage your weight.

Long-Term Commitment: Nutrient-rich, balanced meals are a lifelong approach, not simply a 30-day plan. You're assuring a long-term commitment to a healthy you by including these meals in your usual diet.

Meals that are well-balanced and high in nutrients are a celebration of flavors, wellbeing, and the art of eating healthfully, rather than merely a means of survival. You're not only feeding your body when you accept these meals as an essential component of your everyday routine; you're also strengthening your resolve to long-term health and a better, happier version of yourself.

Meal Schedules and Shopping Catalogs

Creating a shopping list and a meal plan are effective tools that help you on your path to better health. We will introduce you to the idea of planned meal plans and detailed shopping lists in Week 4 of your 30-Day Weight Loss Challenge. These resources can change the way you think about nutrition and grocery shopping. Here's how:

Effective Nutrition Planning: Meal plans give you a productive way to set up your daily snacks and meals. They save you time and effort by taking the guesswork out of choosing what to eat and when.

Rich in nutrients and well-balanced: Meal plans with a structured format are made to be both of these things. They control your calorie consumption while making sure you get a wide range of vital nutrients.

Meal plans place a strong emphasis on portion control since it helps you stay within a healthy weight range and prevents overeating. Every meal is thoughtfully portioned to support your objectives.

Variety and Enjoyment: A range of flavors, foods, and cuisines are included in these plans. This diversity guarantees that you receive a wide range of nutrients and also makes your meals interesting.

Adaptable to Preferences: Meal plans are adaptable to your dietary requirements and preferences. The plans can be customized to meet your needs, regardless of whether you follow a vegetarian, vegan, or gluten-free diet.

Streamlined Grocery Shopping: The shopping lists that go with products are made to make the process of buying groceries easier. They save you from having to make numerous journeys to the grocery store by listing every component you'll need for your meal plan.

Food waste can be decreased by adhering to planned meal plans and the shopping lists that go along with them. You make effective use of the components and only purchase what you require.

Time and Money Savings: Well-organized shopping lists and effective meal planning help you save both. When you have a thorough shopping list and a well-organized meal plan, you're less inclined to eat out or get takeout.

Long-Term Health Commitment: Creating meal planning and shopping lists is a method for committing to a healthier you for the long term, not only for the length of the challenge. You can make sure that you keep up your health and well-being by integrating these resources into your daily routine.

The goal of well-organized shopping lists and structured meal plans is to make nutrition approachable, pleasurable, and manageable. They assist you in taking charge of your nutrition, organizing your buying, and making sure that your meals complement your health objectives. By utilizing these tools, you may prepare for a lifetime of health and happiness rather than just your meals.

CHAPTER FOUR

Stories of Success

Success stories are a vital and motivating component of your path to better health. We tell you these stories in Week 4 of your

30-Day Weight Loss Challenge, not just as inspirational tales of success but also as proof that you, too, can reach your wellness and health objectives.

Success stories serve as a reminder that everyone has the capacity to make meaningful changes in their life. They are living examples of how you may overcome obstacles and reach your wellness and health objectives with perseverance, commitment, and the appropriate techniques. Remember that you too may write your own success story—a narrative of perseverance and metamorphosis on the road to a better, happier version of yourself—as you read and consider these experiences.

Actual Metamorphoses: Motivational Tales of Success

Real-life transformations provide the strongest proof of the value of commitment, perseverance, and pursuing one's goals in the field of health and wellness. This section contains a number of incredible real-life makeovers that will undoubtedly speak to your own needs, goals, problems, and objectives. These aren't just anecdotes; they serve as real-life examples of how the 30-Day Weight Loss Challenge may result in significant improvements and a revitalized sense of wellbeing. Here are just a few of the amazing changes you can expect:

1. Getting Rid of the Weight Battle: Sarah's Path to Wellbeing

Introducing Sarah, who, like many others, was caught in a vicious cycle of weight gain and reduction. Her narrative details her incredible journey away from the frustration of yo-yo dieting and toward accepting long-term adjustments to her food and exercise routine. Sarah's recovery serves as evidence of what may happen when someone takes a thoughtful, balanced approach to wellbeing.

2. Regaining Happiness with Exercise: John's Transformational Fitness Story

Accompany John on a life-changing adventure that centers around a little but significant adjustment: incorporating consistent exercise into his routine. John's narrative, which began with him leading a sedentary lifestyle, demonstrates the healing potential of regular exercise and how it can give one access to previously unattainable levels of vitality and energy.

3. Revealing the Inner Calm: Sarah's Journey from Stress to Peace:

Sarah's story is representative of many people who find it difficult to juggle the responsibilities of their families, careers, and personal care. As she learns how to manage her stress and incorporate self-care and mindfulness practices to find peace in her everyday life, her transformation becomes more evident.

4. Awakening by Rest: Mark's Path to Sleep Restoration

Mark's narrative highlights the often overlooked significance of restful sleep for general health and wellbeing. Mark had increased vitality, mental clarity, and a more vibrant existence when he changed his sleeping patterns and recovered healing sleep.

Weight Loss Warriors: Motivational True Tales of Success

This section contains a collection of weight reduction success stories from people who overcame a wide range of obstacles, such as emotional eating and sedentary lives. These stories illustrate the range of encounters and successes that can be had when pursuing wellness.

Honoring Milestones: The Participants' Little Steps and Great Triumphs

This chapter is devoted to honoring the accomplishments of fellow travelers who have reached noteworthy turns in their journey. Their accomplishments, no matter how big or small, serve as a mirror for your amazing potential and the opportunities that lie ahead.

Pearls of Wisdom from the Community: Participants' Thoughts and Lessons

Give yourself over to the voices of people in the community who openly discuss their experiences, failures, and life lessons learned. Their insights provide a special fusion of viewpoints and useful advice that can enlighten your own journey.

These real-life makeovers are not fantastical stories; rather, they are tangible illustrations of what is possible when willpower, introspection, and wellbeing come together. They provide unquestionable proof that your wellness journey may result in significant, life-changing improvement because they profoundly connect with your needs, goals, problems, and objectives. While perusing these inspiring tales of success, keep in mind that they are a mirror of your own boundless potential, just waiting to be unlocked on your journey toward a better, more contented version of yourself.

Participants' Thoughts and Lessons: Group Wisdom for Your Wellness Journey

You'll find a wealth of knowledge and advice kindly provided by other 30-Day Weight Loss Challenge participants in this section. Their stories, setbacks, and victories are more than simply anecdotes; they are evidence of the combined experience of those who have traveled a route comparable to your own, experiencing similar needs, goals, problems, and wants. Here are a few of the priceless revelations and lessons you can expect:

1. The Power of Consistency: A lot of people emphasize how crucial it is to maintain constant healthy practices. They stress that major long-term changes in weight, fitness, and general well-being can result from relatively modest daily efforts.

2. Adopting Mindful Eating: A number of people draw attention to the life-changing potential of mindful eating techniques. They discuss how their relationship with food was improved and overeating was reduced by being present throughout meals, appreciating every bite, and paying attention to hunger cues.

3. Finding Harmony in Everyday Life: Juggling job, family, and health is a frequent struggle. Participants provide useful tips for creating a peaceful daily schedule that supports mental and physical health, such as time management methods and setting limits.

4. Coping with Cravings and Emotional Eating: Participants discuss their methods for managing emotional eating, which is a common challenge. Their courses offer advice on overcoming urges, from recognizing triggers to locating healthy emotional outlets.

5. The Transformational Power of Exercise: Many participants emphasize the advantages of engaging in regular physical activity. They talk about how they found joy in moving, created a fitness regimen that works for them, and saw amazing improvements in both their physical and mental well-being.

6. The Function of Accountability and Support: A number of individuals stress the significance of support networks. They talk about how being part of a community, getting professional help, or having an accountability partner were essential to their journey toward wellness.

7. How to Handle Setbacks and Plateaus: Any trip will inevitably encounter setbacks and plateaus.

Participants share their perspectives on how they overcame these obstacles by changing their tactics, remaining driven, and adopting an optimistic outlook.

8. Putting Self-Compassion Into Practice: A common theme among the participants is self-compassion. They emphasize the value of treating oneself with kindness, particularly in trying times, and share how their self-compassion has enabled them to keep going.

9. Milestone Celebration: Discussion participants emphasize the value of acknowledging all accomplishments, no matter how minor. They discuss how commemorating achievements kept them motivated and served as a reminder of their advancements.

10. Accepting a Lifelong endeavor: One frequent theme is the idea that wellbeing is a lifelong endeavor. Participants emphasize that creating long-lasting, sustainable behaviors is the secret to long-term health and pleasure, and that the 30-Day Weight Loss Challenge is just the start.

These realizations and teachings are more than just words on a page; they reflect the collective experience of those who have started along the same path to wellbeing as you. They are mirrors of shared wants, problems, aspirations, and needs. Recall that the combined knowledge and experiences of your peers can serve as a source of inspiration and guidance for you as you forge your own, individual path toward a happier, healthier version of yourself.

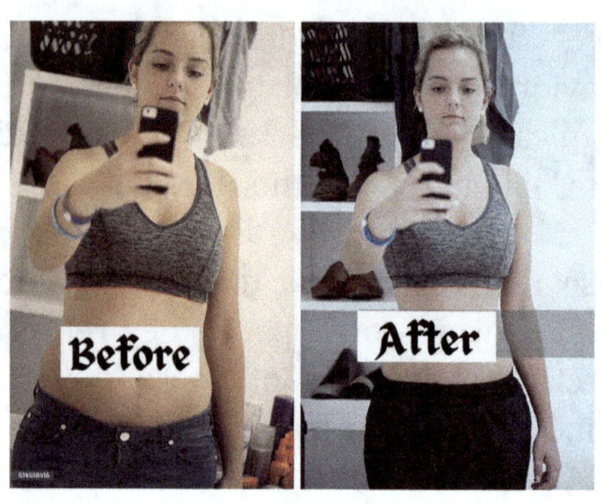
Before
After

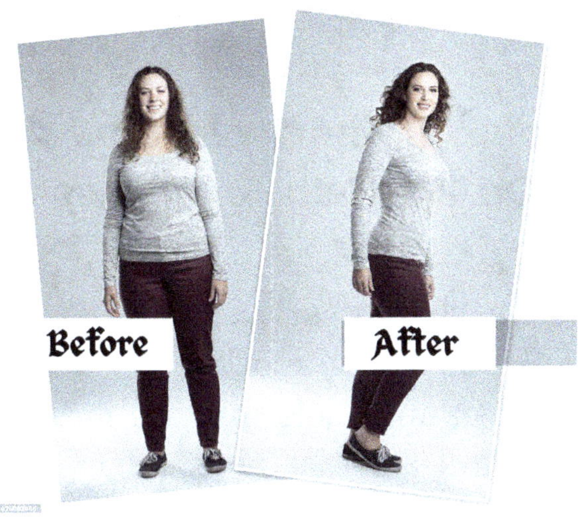

Before
After

CHAPTER FIVE

Resources And Tools: Your Allies On The Path To Wellness

The sixth chapter of your 30-Day Weight Loss Challenge unlocks a wealth of information and tools that are meant to be your faithful allies as you embark on your path to a healthier you. These tools are more than simply things; they are allies to help you, mentors to enlighten you, and instruments to empower you.

Your tools and resources are active agents on your path, not only things or ideas. Consider them your allies, there to help, encourage, and stand with you. Your route to wellness is strengthened, your goals are within grasp, and your trip is enhanced with the prospect of being a happier and healthier version of yourself when these allies are by your side.

Suggested Applications and Resources: Your Digital Armoury for Well-Being

Your digital toolkit for wellness is unveiled in the section on suggested apps and resources in your 30-Day Weight Loss Challenge. These tools are more than simply applications; they're virtual allies that are prepared to support and enable you as you embark on your path to better health. Here's how using these suggested tools and apps might change the way you think about wellness and health:

Accurate Tracking: Suggested applications provide accurate tracking of your daily activities, including steps taken and caloric consumed. They give you up-to-date information on your development, enabling you to modify your wellness plan.

Food Planning Made Simple: Making a balanced, nutrient-dense food plan is made easier with meal planning applications. They provide shopping lists for quick and easy supermarket excursions and provide a large selection of recipes that you may modify to fit your dietary restrictions.

Workout Wizards: Your pocket-sized personal trainer is available through fitness applications. They provide video demos, coach you through exercises, and monitor your progress. It's easy to workout according to your fitness level and schedule using these applications.

Apps for mindfulness and meditation provide a tranquil getaway from the demands of daily life. They offer techniques for stress management and enhancing mental clarity, as well as guided meditation sessions and deep breathing exercises.

Health and Wellness Monitoring: You may monitor important parameters like blood pressure, weight, and sleep quality with apps made specifically for this purpose. They assist you in closely monitoring your general state of well-being.

Nutrition Analysis: Your personal nutrition counselors are apps that perform nutritional analysis. They let you input recipes, scan barcodes, and determine the nutritional value of the food you eat. These apps support you in making well-informed food decisions.

Community and Support: Connecting to wellness communities through apps gives you access to a network of people who can help you. They let you celebrate victories together, exchange stories about your path, and receive guidance from others.

Educational Resources: Apps that give users access to educational materials function similarly to portable libraries. They provide articles, videos, and e-books to help you learn more about exercise, nutrition, and health.

Goal-Setting and Progress-Tracking Apps: These apps help you create clear targets, monitor your progress, and maintain accountability for your wellness goals.

Motivational Information: A lot of wellness applications provide inspirational quotations, testimonies, and success stories as well as other motivational information. They act as continual reminders of your abilities and your dedication to well-being.

Customization to Meet Specific Needs: The majority of these apps offer a great deal of customization, so you may make your experience meet your own requirements and tastes. You have the ability to customize your wellness path, set goals, and change settings.

Data security and privacy are given top priority by trustworthy wellness apps. Your digital journey is secret and secure since your health and personal information are safeguarded.

These suggested tools and applications are more than simply icons on your screen; they serve as doorsways to a happier and healthier version of yourself. They provide you the tools, convenience, and direction to take charge of your journey toward health and wellness. Keep in mind that you have allies in the digital world who will help you along the journey as you maneuver through this arsenal.

Further Reading and Sources: Increasing Your Understanding of Wellness

The section on supplementary reading and references in your 30-Day Weight Loss Challenge is a treasure trove of information inside the vast terrain of the program. These materials are your guides to a greater comprehension of health and wellbeing, not just a list of references. The following additional reading and resources can help you become more knowledgeable and confident in your quest for better health:

Extensive Reading and References: These resources provide a framework for delving deeper into issues pertaining to wellness, fitness, nutrition, and health. They provide you the chance to delve further into topics that catch your attention.

Evidence-Based Knowledge: A lot of these resources are based on professional judgment and scientific studies. They are trustworthy providers of knowledge based on evidence, assisting you in making well-informed decisions regarding your well-being.

Comprehensive Insights: Research papers, books, and articles frequently offer thorough insights into particular facets of wellness and health. They provide a comprehensive perspective on subjects, assisting you in developing a well-rounded knowledge.

Specialized Knowledge: Writers of some references are authorities in their respective fields. They impart their specific knowledge to you, giving you useful advice and tactics that are the result of years of experience.

Practical Guidance: There are references available that provide useful advice and direction. They provide you the ability to apply the knowledge to your everyday life by breaking down difficult ideas into manageable steps.

Motivation and mentality: A wealth of resources explore the psychological dimensions of health and wellbeing, assisting you in cultivating the appropriate mentality and sustaining your motivation as you proceed.

Historical and Cultural Viewpoints: A few readings discuss wellness practices from historical and cultural angles. They provide insightful examples of how many societies have viewed health and wellness over time.

Cookbooks and Recipe Collections: Cookbooks and recipe collections resemble culinary manuals. They help you make healthy eating enjoyable by providing an abundance of tasty and nutritious meal ideas.

Case Studies and Success Stories: Sources that contain case studies and success stories provide actual accounts of people who have reached their wellness and health objectives. Stories from these sources provide inspiration and practical insights..

Encouragement and Support: Reading about the experiences of others might provide a feeling of encouragement and support. It serves as a reminder that you're not the only one pursuing wellness and good health.

Community and Connection: You'll frequently find a group of people who share your enthusiasm for health and wellness through books, articles, and references. They offer chances to network with people who share your objectives.

Updates and Current Trends: You can stay current on the most recent developments in the fields of wellness and health by consulting the references. They make sure you may get the most recent data available.

These suggested readings and sources are more than just words on paper—they're your passes to a more comprehensive grasp of wellness and health. Keep in mind that these tools are there to empower you, expand your knowledge, and help you on your path to being a better and healthier version of yourself as you explore them.

CHAPTER SIX

Conclusion: Your Ongoing Journey To Wellness

As you approach the last chapter of your 30-Day Weight Loss Challenge, remember that this is a fresh start rather than the end of the journey. The end serves as a reminder to keep moving forward on your path to wellbeing rather than a farewell. Your path to wellness is evidence of your dedication to happiness, balance, and good health. Keep in mind that the ending is only the beginning of a route that leads far into the future as you read it. Your lifelong path to a better, happier version of yourself will be accompanied by your dedication, the information you've acquired, and the community you've formed.

Examining Your 30-Day Experience: The Influence of Positive Self-Talk

As your 30-Day Weight Loss Challenge draws to a close, it's important to pause and consider the incredible trip you've already undertaken. This process of reflection is more than simply a step; it's a transforming one that encourages thankfulness, self-acceptance, and the realization that you are the creator of your own well-being. Here are some tips for strengthening your 30-day journey to a healthy you:

Acknowledging Your Success: When you think back, acknowledge the successes—no matter how minor—that you've had over the course of these 30 days. Your strength and tenacity are demonstrated by your capacity to develop and achieve goals.

Accepting Progress: Consider the strides you've accomplished. Maybe you've started an exercise regimen, made better dietary choices, or shed some weight. Recognize the efforts you've made to reach your wellness objectives.

Learning from Difficulties: Difficulties are chances for development rather than failures. Think back on the difficulties you've faced and be grateful for the lessons they've taught you. You will find these lessons useful in your continued travels.

Expressing gratitude for the support you have received during this challenge from friends, family, and the community. Thanking them for their assistance not only recognizes their contribution but also fortifies your relationship.

Recognizing Your Resilience: You have probably experienced setbacks and periods of self-doubt along the way. Think about your resilience—your capacity to overcome obstacles and carry on with your quest for well-being.

This is an opportunity to cultivate self-appreciation. Recognize your dedication to improving yourself and the actions you've taken to put your health and wellbeing first.

Honoring Consistency: Advancement is frequently predicated on consistency. Celebrate your dedication to consistency, whether it is in the form of mindfulness exercises, a regular workout schedule, or better eating habits.

Strengthening a Positive Attitude: A positive attitude can be strengthened by your reflection. It serves as a reminder that you are capable of bringing about change and that you can achieve your objectives.

Viewing Wellness as a Journey: This contemplation emphasizes that achieving wellness is a journey rather than a goal. It motivates you to see happiness and health as a continuous process.

Creating New Objectives: Think about the objectives you wish to accomplish in the future while you reflect. These could be brand-new ambitions or an expansion of your present ones. Creating fresh goals for your path keeps it interesting and active.

Acknowledging the Power inside: Thinking back on your experience helps you recognize the ability to bring about change inside yourself. Realizing that you are in control of your wellness path is empowering.

Creating a Gratitude-Driven Attitude: Gratitude is a powerful emotion. Think back on the abundance in your life, such as the chance to better yourself, the availability of resources, and the relationships that provide support.

Proceeding on the Journey: This contemplation marks not a conclusion but an inception. It marks the beginning of a path toward lifelong wellness. You're prepared for what's coming because of your self-awareness and the lessons you've learned.

Looking back on your 30-day adventure is a celebration of your development, tenacity, and dedication to bettering yourself. As you reflect, keep in mind that each step you've taken has brought you closer to becoming a better, healthier version of yourself. Your journey is not limited to just 30 days; rather, it is a continuous road that offers countless chances for growth and wellbeing.

Advancing Toward a Healthier Way of Life: Overcoming the Obstacle

When your 30-Day Weight Loss Challenge comes to a conclusion, it's time to focus on creating a healthier lifestyle that will last far longer than this short challenge. Choosing to live a better lifestyle going ahead involves realizing that your journey to wellness is a lifetime commitment rather than just continuing the struggle. Here's how to welcome this change with purpose and enthusiasm:

Sustainable Habits: Making the shift to a healthier lifestyle necessitates substituting short-term adjustments with long-term routines. Recognize the improvements you've made during the challenge and incorporate them into your everyday activities. Developing improved food habits, consistent exercise routines, or mindfulness exercises should become second nature to you.

Goal-setting: Creating fresh objectives is essential to your ongoing development. Think about the long- and short-term goals you have in mind. These objectives can include reducing weight, getting fitter, reducing stress, or focusing on any other area of wellbeing that is important to you. Establishing clear, attainable goals helps you stay motivated and concentrated.

Conscious Decisions: The foundation of a healthy lifestyle is consciousness. Pay attention to your diet, your exercise regimen, and your stress-reduction techniques. Make decisions that support your values and wellness objectives.

Frequent Exercise: Exercise need to be an integral part of your daily routine.Look for activities that fit your schedule and that you enjoy doing. Regular physical activity, whether it be through team sports, weight training, yoga, or daily walks, is essential for good health.

Balanced Nutrition: Keep putting an emphasis on maintaining a balanced diet. Make entire food choices, eat a range of fruits and vegetables, and watch how much you eat. For optimal energy and overall health, keep your intake of macronutrients (fats, proteins, and carbohydrates) in balance.

Stress Management: Although stress is inevitable in life, how you handle it can have a big impact on your well-being. Maintain your stress-reduction regimen by doing deep breathing exercises, meditation, or indulging in enjoyable hobbies.

Sleep Hygiene: Getting enough good sleep is crucial to general health. Make sure you obtain the recommended amount of sleep each night, stick to a regular sleep pattern, and make your surroundings favorable to rest.

Support and Community: Continue to be involved in the groups you've formed during the challenge. The friendship and support of others who have similar values can be very beneficial for continued accountability and inspiration.

Educational Development: Keep learning about wellness and health. To increase your knowledge, read books, articles, and conduct research. Participate in seminars, workshops, and courses to expand your knowledge on particular wellness-related subjects.

Flexibility and Adaptability: Since life is full of surprises, adopting a healthier lifestyle may present unanticipated difficulties. Adopt a flexible and adaptive mindset in your strategy. Acquire the ability to modify your tactics and overcome obstacles.

Self-compassion: Treat yourself with kindness as you travel. Recognize that it's OK to make mistakes or doubt yourself occasionally. Be kind to yourself and see these times as a chance to improve.

Celebrate Your Milestones: Acknowledge and honor your accomplishments as you go. Acknowledge your accomplishments and make the most of these occasions to inspire you to keep going.

Accept the Journey: Keep in mind that achieving wellbeing is an ongoing endeavor. With excitement, embrace it, for it is a path full of opportunities for self-discovery and ongoing development.

Adopting a healthier lifestyle is merely the next chapter in a book with many unwritten pages; it is not the conclusion. It's a chance to take care of your health, live intentionally, and become the best version of yourself. With great enthusiasm and a strong dedication to your long-term well-being, embrace this change.